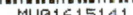

Linda Rector Page
N.D., PhD.

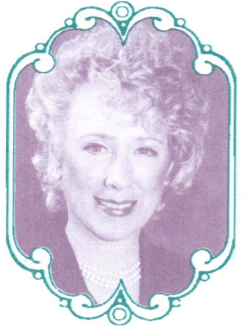

Detoxification
&
Body Cleansing
To Fight Disease

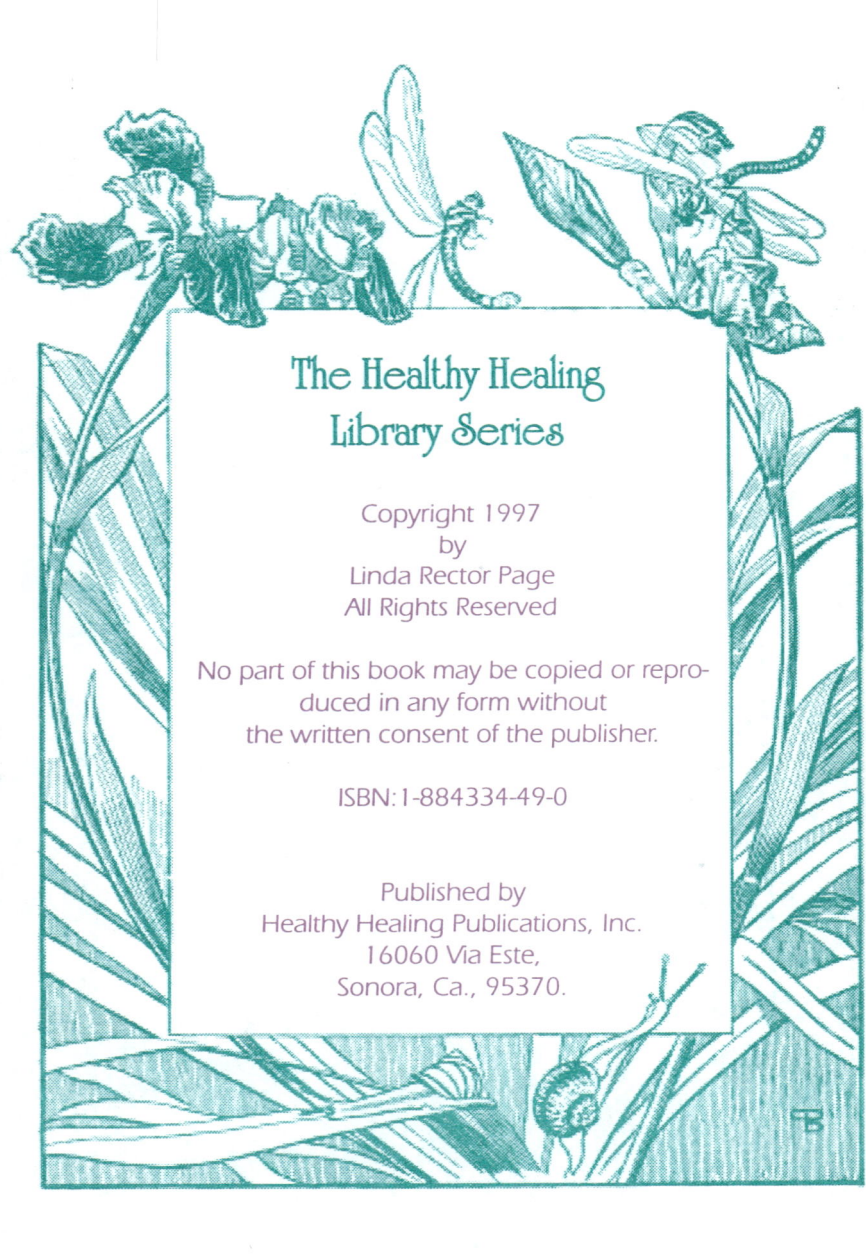

The Healthy Healing Library Series

ISBN:1-884334-49-0

Published by
Healthy Healing Publications, Inc.
16060 Via Este,
Sonora, Ca., 95370.

Table of Contents

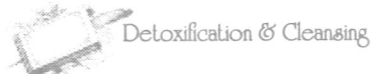

Who Needs To Detoxify?

Detoxification is becoming necessary for everybody. No one can escape the enormous amount of environmental toxins assaulting us in the world today. No one is immune to every unhealthy lifestyle choice.

How do we remain healthy in a destructive environment? There's no doubt about it. Americans are immersed in synthetic, often toxic substances. Every system of the body is affected, from deep level tissue damage to sensory deterioration.

Today, people are exposed to chemicals on an unprecedented scale. More than 2 million synthetic substances are known, 25,000 are added each year, and over 30,000 are produced on a commercial scale. Only a tiny fraction are ever tested for toxicity, and many come to us on the winds from developing countries that have few safeguards in place.

Many chemicals are so widely spread that we are unaware of them. But they work their way into our bodies faster than they can be eliminated, and are causing allergies and addictions in record numbers. Industrial chemicals and their pollutant by-products, pesticides and additives in our foods, heavy metals, anesthetics, residues from all kinds of drugs, and environmental hormones are trapped within the human body in greater concentrations than at any other point in history. And these things don't even count the secondary smoke, caffeine and alcohol overloads, or daily stress that are an increasing part of our lives.

Because the molecular structure of many chemical carcinogens interacts with human DNA, long term exposure can result in metabolic and genetic alteration that affects cell growth, behavior and immune response. New research by the World Health Organization implicates toxic environmental chemicals in 60 to 80% of many cancers. Studies also link pesticides and pollutants to hormone dysfunctions, psychological disorders, birth defects, still births and now breast cancer.

The wide variety of toxic substances means that toxic matter saturates every body system; anti-oxidants and minerals in vital body cells and fluids are reduced, immune defenses are thrown out of balance. Vitality is overwhelmed and eventually disease begins. Circumstances like this have become the prime factor in today's immune compromised diseases like candidiasis, lupus, fibromyalgia, chronic fatigue syndrome, and cancer.

Chemical oxidation is the other process that affects body degeneration and allows disease. The oxygen that "rusts" and ages us also triggers free radical activity, a destructive cascade of incomplete molecules that damages DNA and other cell components. And if you didn't have a reason to reduce your fat intake before, oxygen combines with fats in body storage cells to speed up the free radical deterioration process.

I believe we are in a paradigm shift in humanity's time on the planet. For millions of years, the Earth has controlled its own destiny. But humans have risen in intelligence and command, to challenge the Earth - even the universe and the stars. In the last few decades we have become dangerously able to harm the health of our planet, even to the point of making it uninhabitable for life. We must develop further and take even larger steps... not the steps of rule and challenge, but those of cooperation and support.

The analogy to atomic power is clear. Fission is great, but fusion is greater. The well-being of the world depends on the **alliance** of mankind and the Earth together, to save it all for us all. It starts with ourselves.

How do you know if you need to detoxify? Almost everybody does. It's one of the best ways to remain healthy in a chemical-laced environment. Not one of us is immune to environmental toxins, and most of us can't escape to a remote, pristine habitat. But we can take a closer look at our own air, water and food, and keep it as clean as possible. We can take positive steps to keep our own body cleansing systems in good working order. And we can keep a watchful eye on the politics that control our environment. Legislation on health and the environment follows two pathways in America today... the influence of business and politics, and the demands of the people for a healthy environment and responsible stewardship of the Earth.

Our bodies are clearly created as self-cleaning, self-healing mechanisms. Internal detoxification is an ongoing process performed on a daily basis. Just as our hearts beat nonstop and our lungs breathe automatically, so our metabolic processes continually dispose of wastes and poisons. Detoxification is the body's natural process of eliminating or neutralizing toxins, by the liver, kidneys, colon, lungs and skin. If you keep immune response high, elimination regular, circulation sound, and stress under control, your body can handle a great deal of toxicity and regularly prevent disease. Yet, organs that were once completely capable of detoxification may be so overloaded that they become unable to purify us of the daily poisons that assault us. So poisons build up in our systems, and eventually result in disease.

In the past, detoxification was used either clinically for recovering alcoholics and drug addicts, or individually as a once-a-year mild "spring cleaning" for general health. Today, a regular detoxification program two or three times a year can make a big difference in the way your body performs. It might be the missing link for preventing chronic diseases like cancer, candida, chronic fatigue, arthritis, diabetes and obesity.

Most people eat too much animal protein, fat, caffeine, alcohol, and chemicalized foods that inhibit optimum cell function. Even if your diet is good, a cleanse can restore body vitality against environmental toxins. **Detoxification supports both health, and the quality of our lives.**

Here are some signs that you may need to detoxify:
- If you get frequent, unexplained headaches or back pain,
- if you have chronic respiratory problems, sinus problems or asthma,
- if you have abnormal body odor, bad breath or coated tongue,
- if you have food allergies, poor digestion, or constipation with chronic intestinal bloating, or unexplained weight gain over 10 pounds.
- if you have brittle nails and hair, psoriasis, or adult acne.
- if you have joint pain, or arthritis,
- if you are depressed and irritable, and always out of energy,
- if you have unusually poor memory and chronic insomnia.

Here are some of the benefits you can expect from a body cleanse:
- Your digestive tract is cleansed of accumulated waste and fermenting bacteria.
- Liver, kidney and blood purification take place, impossible under ordinary eating patterns.
- Mental clarity is enhanced, impossible under chemical overload.
- Dependency on habit-forming substances, such as sugar, caffeine, nicotine, alcohol and drugs, is reduced as the blood stream is purified.
- Bad eating habits are often turned around, and the stomach has a chance to reduce to normal size for weight control.

Herbs are effective for a broad spectrum of body cleansing goals.

Herbs, particularly organically grown herbs, are rich in food-source minerals, vitamins, amino acids, and enzyme precursors. Herbs provide concentrated, whole food nutrition that becomes part of the body to stimulate cleansing, fuel regrowth, and build resistance to disease. Herbs are unique among therapeutic media in these abilities, in a way that drugs, or even partitioned substances like vitamins are not. They work with the body's own action as a source of life and growth. This is the key to their success as natural medicines.

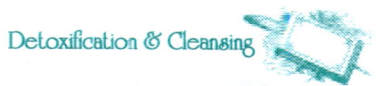

**A good detox program should be in three stages:
1) Cleansing, 2) Rebuilding, and 3) Maintaining
Herbs, in their abundance of diversity and in the specific
nature of their activity are ideally suited to these tasks.**

Here's how to tailor a cleansing program to your specific needs:
First consider what you really need to do. A live food, juice and herb cleanse literally picks up dead matter from the body and carries it away. Cleansing also helps release hormone secretions that stimulate immune response, and encourage a disease-preventing environment.
•Do you need a mild spring body cleansing?
•Do you need to eliminate drug residues?
•Does your body need to normalize after a disease or hospital stay?
•Do you need a jump start for a healing program?
•Do you need a detox program for a serious health problem?

Next, consider the time factor. How long can you give out of your busy lifestyle to focus on a cleansing program? 24 hours, 2 or 3 days, or up to ten days? It's important to allot your time ahead of time, so that all the processes of the cleanse can be completed.
The second part of a good cleansing program is rebuilding healthy tissue and restoring body energy. This phase allows the body's regulating powers to become active with obstacles removed, so it can rebuild at optimum levels. A rebuilding diet emphasizes fresh, simply prepared foods. It should be very low in fat, with little dairy, and no fried food. Avoid alcohol, caffeine, tobacco, and sugars. Avoid meats except fish and sea foods. Herbal support should be included for specific needs.
The final part of a good cleansing program is keeping your body clean and toxin-free - very important after all the hard work of detoxification. Modifying lifestyle habits to include high quality nutrition from both food and herbal sources is the key to a strong resistant body. A diet for health maintenance should rely heavily on fresh fruits and vegetables. A personalized group of supplements and herbal aids, as well as exercise and relaxation techniques, should be included.

After a cleanse, the body starts rebalancing, energy levels rise physically, psychologically and sexually, and creativity begins to expand. You start feeling like a "different person" - and of course you are.
Your outlook and attitude change, because through cleansing and improved diet, your actual cell make-up has changed.
You really are what you eat.

Do you always have to fast?

Fasting is used as a detoxification method because it can rapidly increase the elimination of wastes and enhance the healing process. One of the world's oldest known therapies, fasting has been used regularly up to modern times by naturopaths and herbalists as part of a healing course for a wide range of diseases, both physiological and psychological. The sound healing principles of fasting have long been known; stress is removed from essential organs and body processes so that healing and rebuilding can take place, while non-essential fatty and muscle tissue is used for fuel.

A few days without solid food can be a refreshing and enlightening experience about your lifestyle. I like to think of fasting as a technique that takes your body back to the starting gate, so that you don't run with a dirty engine or drive with the brakes on.

A short fast increases awareness as well as energy availability for elimination. Your body will become easier to "hear." It can tell you what foods and diet are right for your needs via cravings, such as a desire for protein foods, or B vitamins or minerals, for example.
Like a "cell phone call," body cravings are natural bio-feedback.

Fasting works by self-digestion. During a cleanse, the body decomposes and burns only the substances and tissues that are damaged, diseased or unneeded, such as abscesses, tumors, excess fat deposits, and congestive wastes. Even a relatively short fast accelerates elimination, often causing dramatic changes as masses of accumulated waste are expelled.

You will be very aware of this if you experience the short period of headaches, fatigue, body odor, bad breath, diarrhea or mouth sores that commonly accompany accelerated elimination. Most people encountering these reactions realize that their bodies have thrown off serious toxins because their digestion and many obvious organ functions usually improve right away.

With years of experience in fasting programs of all types, I am convinced that a moderate 3 to 7 day juice fast is the best way to release toxins from the system. Shorter fasts don't really get to the root of a chronic or major problem. Longer fasts upset body equilibrium more than most people are ready to deal with except in a controlled, clinical situation.

A moderate juice fast with herbal support and green superfoods can bring great advantages by cleansing your body of excess mucous, old fecal matter, trapped cellular, and non-food wastes, and by "cleaning the pipes" of systemic sludge such as inorganic mineral deposits.

Different Types of Detoxification Programs

There are several effective types of cleanses you can tailor to your specific needs. Unless you are addressing a serious illness, or recovering from a long course of drugs or chemical therapy, consider a detoxification cleanse twice a year, especially in the spring, summer or early fall, when sunlight and natural vitamin D can offer the body an extra boost.

A mild "spring cleanse" is important in a healthy lifestyle. Even though we may exercise during the winter to keep trim, most people still feel at an energy low during cold seasons. And there is no question, much to the dismay of many of us, that fall and winter are difficult times of the year to control body weight. Our bodies still reflect the ancient cold weather need to harbor more fat for warmth and survival. And cold weather prompts people to consume heavier, fattier, comfort foods.

In the days when people were closer to nature than we are today, the great majority farmed the land from spring to fall, and lived lives of demanding physical labor. Winter was a time of inactivity, with a natural tendency towards rest. Food supplies stored in the autumn lost much of their nutrition. Even in modern times, many days without sunshine and vitamin D mean that our bodies are less able to utilize nutrients properly.

Winter weather illnesses like colds and flu leave us with an accumulation of toxins. Heavy winter clothing, especially thick waterproof coats, hinder deep breathing and perspiration, and contribute to clogged body functions. When spring finally arrives, our metabolism livens up. Warmer weather tends to lower appetites and prompts more activity and movement. It's easier to stimulate cleansing processes. New, green food sources, with their metabolism-stimulating effects, abound from the first tender shoots of herbs and leafy vegetables. Cleansing, anti-oxidant-rich herbs promote a feeling of new life and restored well-being. It's time to go on a spring cleanse.

A "spring cleaning" is actually a very light diet, focusing on digestion and the intestines to help eliminate accumulated wastes, and improve body functions. A good length for a spring cleanse is 2 or 3 days or long weekend. A weekend is enough time to fit comfortably into most people's lives, and it doesn't become too stressful on the body. The best way is to start on Friday night with a pre-cleansing salad, then follow with a cleansing diet like the one in HEALTHY HEALING or COOKING FOR HEALTHY HEALING by Linda Rector Page, and end with a light Monday morning fruit bowl. Amplify the purifying effect with a stimulating, circulation bath or a hot SEAWEED BATH (see page 29).

A three to ten day healing program cleanse focuses on more ambitious detoxification, and it's often a good choice for those who are addressing serious health problems. I recommend using this type of detox for only up to 10 days at any one time. Cleansing for more than ten days may dredge up deep seated toxins (like DDT) that, when released can result in concentrated amounts that the body can't handle, especially if it is in a weakened state. Body stress may also increase to the point where healing stops, defeating the purpose of the cleanse. If you want to go on a longer detox schedule, break it up into several segments of 7 to 10 days each, and adjust your target areas for specific health problems.

A long 4 day weekend is an ideal starting time for many people. Remember, a detox and cleanse is just the beginning of your healing program. Don't overdo it. Efficient, yet gentle herbal aids to cleansing can go a long way to accelerating the process, and shortening the time frame. As with other cleanses, a longer detox involves a pre-fasting meal, aimed at tee-ing your body up for increased elimination. It moves into a juice fast accompanied with herbal supplements, plenty of water, some exercise and stress-reduction techniques. See **HEALTHY HEALING or COOKING FOR HEALTHY HEALING by Linda Rector Page** for complete details of this type of moderate cleanse.

A 24 hour cleanse can be a good answer if you need a cleanse, but your busy life won't allow you to set aside even a few days. People have busy lives. Even a short cleanse seems like too much time.

"Beginning" is usually the hardest part of a cleanse. You have to set aside a block of time, gather all the ingredients for your diet, alter eating times and patterns; in essence change your lifestyle and that of those you live with for a while. This is very difficult to do for many people, and can delay a needed program.

A 24-hour detox is a juice and herbal tea cleanse that lets you go on with your normal activities, yet still "jump start" a healing program. Even though it's quick, without the depth of vegetable juices needed for a chronic problem, it's often enough, is definitely better than no cleanse at all, and it will make a difference in the speed of healing. Even if your program is only going to consist of lifestyle changes aimed at better health, a 24 hour cleanse can point you in the right direction.

Here is the 24 hour cleanse:

•Start the night before with a green leafy salad to give your bowels a good sweeping. Dry brush your skin before you go to bed to open your pores for the night's cleansing eliminations.

•Then take the next 24 hours for fresh juices, pure water, and a long walk during the day.

On rising: take an 8-oz. glass of water with 2 squeezed lemons and 1TB. maple syrup.

Midmorning: take a glass of cranberry juice from concentrate.

Lunch: take a glass of apple juice, or add a superfood green drink blend to apple juice. I recommend an energy green drink like this:

RICE PROTEIN, BARLEY GRASS AND SPROUTS, ALFALFA LEAF & SPROUTS, BEE POLLEN, ACEROLA CHERRY, OAT & QUINOA SPROUTS, APPLE PECTIN, SIBERIAN GINSENG, SARSAPARILLA, SPIRULINA, CHLORELLA, DANDELION, DULSE, LICORICE RT., GOTU KOLA. (SA - 8150)

Midafternoon: take a cup of tea that provides food-source vitamins, minerals and enzymes to help in the effort of cleansing and purifying. I recommend a cleansing and purifying tea that looks like this:

RED CLOVER, HAWTHORN, ALFALFA, NETTLES, WHITE SAGE, HORSETAIL, ECHINACEA RT, MILK THISTLE SD., PAU D'ARCO, GOTU KOLA, LEMONGRASS, BLUE MALVA, YERBA SANTA. (CD - 5120)

Dinner: take a glass of papaya/pineapple juice to enhance enzyme production, or another glass of apple juice with 1 rounded tablespoon of your favorite green superfood mix.

Before bed: have a cup of mint tea, or MISO soup, or a warming tonic for mind and body such as the meditation tea offered here:

CARDAMOM, CINNAMON, CLOVES, PEPPERCORNS, FENNEL SD., GINGER RT. (RX-5840) for relaxation and strength the next day.

•The next morning: break your fast with fresh fruits and yogurt. Eat light, raw foods during the day, and have a simple, low fat dinner.

•Take a seaweed or mineral bath in the morning and one before you go to bed. Add some favorite beauty/cleansing treatments like a facial, a pedicure, manicure and deep hair conditioning during your bath. Get a full eight hours of rest that night.

A 7 day brown rice cleanse is a good option to a juice cleanse. It's based on macrobiotic principles, and is effective for dropping a few quick pounds and balancing the body when you're feeling energy low or out-of-sorts. It's simple, easy to take, and easy to fit in with your lifestyle.

•Simply drink 2 to 3 glasses of mixed fresh vegetable juices throughout the day whenever you like, or take 1 rounded tablespoon of your favorite green superfood mixed into water or a juice. Don't eat any solid food during the day.

•Have steamed brown rice and a blend of mixed vegetables for an early dinner. Have at least a cup of rice and several cups of vegetables.

•Add non-fat seasonings to your taste. NO butter or oil dressings.

That's all there is to it. Follow this diet for 6 days. Results in weight, body definition and body chemistry change are noticeable almost immediately. You need the six days to set up an ongoing body balance. Then ease yourself into a good, on-going healthy diet. Try not to let the "reward mode" trigger a binge on fats and sugars. Much of the time your body will crave healthy nutrients it needs. You can watch for these. It's interesting!

Detoxification Diets For Specific Body Needs

Colon Elimination Cleanse: *a 3 to 10 day diet:*

A colon elimination cleanse is something most of us need. The bowel and colon are essential to body detoxification. Just like a city, our bodies deteriorate if our sewage systems aren't cared for. The colon and bowel are the depository for all waste material after nutrients have been extracted into the bloodstream. Unless eliminated regularly, decaying food ferments and forms gases and second generation toxins, which release from the bowel into the bloodstream, causing organ dysfunction and accelerated aging. The colon becomes a breeding ground for putrefactive bacteria, viruses, parasites, and pathogenic microbes. Our bodies can tolerate a certain level of contamination, but when that individual level is reached, it is hardly any wonder that up to 90% of all diseases generate from an unclean colon.

Elements causing colon toxicity come from three basic areas:

1) **Slow elimination time.** Slow bowel transit time allows wastes to become rancid, and then recirculate through the body, exposing all body tissues and organs to the toxins, and lowering overall performance of body functions. Bowel transit time for food should be approximately twelve hours. Over 80% of all human ailments, including headaches, skin blemishes, senility, bad breath, fatigue, arthritis and heart disease can be attributed to an overloaded colon. Waste congestion becomes a breeding ground for parasite infestation, too. A recent nationwide survey revealed that one in every six people studied had parasites living somewhere in their bodies.

2) **Synthetic chemicals in food and environmental pollutants.** A clean, strong system metabolizes and excretes many harmful organ-

isms, but when the body is weak or constipated, they become stored as unusable substances. As more and different chemicals enter the body they tend to inter-react with those that are already there, forming second generation chemicals far more harmful than the originals. Evidence in recent years shows that most colon cancer, the second most prevalent cancer in the United States today, is a direct result of accumulated toxins. Colitis, irritable bowel syndrome, diverticulosis, ileitis and Crohn's disease, are all signs of a toxic colon. They're on the rise, too. Over 100,000 Americans have a colostomy every year! An incredible fact.

3) **Poor digestion.** A high fiber, whole foods diet is both cure and prevention for colon elimination problems. Our rich diet of meats, refined foods, salt and sugar, means we get a lot of grease and little fiber Food fiber's importance comes from its ability to move food through the digestive system quickly and easily, but the Standard American Diet causes a glue-y state that can't be efficiently processed by the intestines. You can picture this if you remember the hard paste formed by white flour and water when you were a kid. Foods are simply crammed into the colon and never fully excreted.

It seems like so much media attention has been focused on high fiber foods for so long, that everybody in America would have changed their diet to a more colon-health oriented pattern. This is simply not the case. Most diet attention has been targeted at reducing fat at all costs, often at the expense of a healthy, fiber-rich diet. Even a gentle, gradual change from low fiber, low residue foods helps almost immediately. In fact, a gradual change is better than a sudden, drastic about-face, especially when the colon is inflamed.

The protective level of fiber in the diet is easily measured:
•The stool should be light enough to float.
•Bowel movements should be regular, daily and effortless.
•The stool should be almost odorless, signalling faster bowel transit time.
•There should be no gas or flatulence.
Tip: *Make a mental note of your colon health every time you have a bowel movement to prevent problems.*

What are the signs that you might need a colon cleanse?
Look for reduced immunity, tiredness, coated tongue, bad breath, body odor, mental dullness and sallow skin. If your cholesterol numbers are too high, a colon cleanse increases absorption of cholesterol-lowering foods and also helps you lose colon congestive weight. You can

easily combine a colon cleanse with a cholesterol cleanse. Add a fiber-rich supplement like the one below for easy fiber, appetite suppression, and acidophilus to restore friendly digestive flora:

ORGANIC OAT BRAN, ORGANIC FLAX SEED, PSYLLIUM HUSKS, GUAR GUM, VEGETABLE ACIDOPHILUS, APPLE PECTIN, ACEROLA CHERRY FRUIT, FENNEL SD., HEARTSEASE LF. (CD - 8100)

Here are some brief pointers to give you the best results for your colon cleanse:

✓Bowel elimination problems are often chronic, and may require several rounds of cleansing. I recommend colon cleansing in periods of five days each.

✓Anyone with a sensitive colon should heal the colon before cleansing it. A very gentle herbal formula like the one below would be a good choice. Avoid a colon cleanser that contains senna or psyllium husks if you have a sensitive or irritated bowel. A soothing, peppermint oil combination provides mild, gentle cleansing.

PEPPERMINT, ALOE VERA, SLIPPERY ELM, MARSHMALLOW RT., PAU D'ARCO, WILD YAM, LOBELIA, GINGER RT. (CD - 1560)

✓A colonic irrigation is a good way to start a bowel cleanse. Grapefruit seed extract is very effective, especially if there is colon toxicity along with constipation. (Dilute to 15 to 20 drops in a gallon of water.) Or take a catnip or diluted liquid chlorophyll enema every other night during the cleanse. *Note:* Enemas may be given to children. Use smaller amounts according to size and age. Allow water to enter very slowly; let them expel when they wish.

✓Drink six to eight glasses of water daily during a colon cleanse.

✓Be sure to take a brisk walk for an hour every day to help keep your elimination channels moving.

✓Take several long warm baths during your cleanse. A lower back and pelvis massage and dry skin brushing will help release toxins coming out through the skin.

Herbal combinations provide both cleansing and tonifying activity. The long history of herbal effectiveness for colon and bowel cleansing offers several good choices for your own specific needs.

#1) The following capsule compound encourages evacuation of the bowels by normal peristalsis. Copious amounts of waste are usually released with this formula. It also tonifies and strengthens the entire elimination system. If taken on a three to six month program to rebuild as well as cleanse the bowel area, this remarkable formula can work in three stages: After current waste is released, hard fecal encrustations are loosened, and cellular acids and wastes are passed; then the herbs begin a toning action for the bowel walls to promote healing of old lesions and elasticizing of flaccid diverticula, so that regular peristalsis can be restored. This combination may be used both short and long term, and often works when nothing else has been effective.

BUTTERNUT BARK, CASCARA SAGRADA, TURKEY RHUBARB, PSYLLIUM HUSKS, BARBERRY BK., FENNEL SD., LICORICE, GINGER, IRISH MOSS, CAPSICUM. (CD - 2350)

#2) The following fiber blend formula provides easy-to-take organic plant fiber necessary to regulate and maintain peristalsis. It is a blend of nature's most complete plant fibers with prime enzyme activity to keep the system clean and healthy. A heaping teaspoon, or four capsules in juice at night offer enough soluble fiber for regularity in the morning.

ORGANIC OAT BRAN, FLAX SEED, PSYLLIUM HUSK, GUAR GUM, VEGETABLE ACIDOPHILUS, APPLE PECTIN, ACEROLA CHERRY, FENNEL SEED, GRAPEFRUIT SEED EXTRACT. (CD - 1850)

#3) The following formula is beneficial when a simple herbal laxative is desired, to quickly relieve constipation or to evacuate the bowels before a fast or cleanse. Its nutrients work rapidly to temporarily increase systole/diastole activity in the colon and bowel. It should only be used on a limited basis so that the body is assured of doing its own work.

SENNA LEAF, FENNEL SEED, PAPAYA, PEPPERMINT, GINGER, LEMON BALM, PARSLEY, HIBISCUS, CALENDULA. (CD - 5720)

Note: Drugstore laxatives aren't really body cleansers. They offer only temporary relief, are usually habit-forming, destructive to intestinal membranes and don't even get to the cause of the problem. They enable the bowels to expel debris only because the colon becomes so irritated by the laxative that it expels whatever loose material is around.

After the initial bowel cleansing program, the second part of a colon health system is rebuilding healthy tissue and body energy. When colon health is compromised, constipation is usually a chronic problem. While body cleansing progress can be felt fairly quickly with a colon detox, it takes from three to six months to rebuild bowel and colon elasticity with good systole/diastole action. The rewards of a regular, energetic life are worth it.

See **HEALTHY HEALING** or **COOKING FOR HEALTHY HEALING** by Linda Rector Page for complete diets and details.

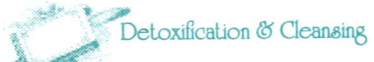

Bladder/Kidney Cleanse: *a 3 to 5 day liquid diet.*

If you have chronic lower back pain, irritated urination, frequent unexplained chills, fever, or nausea, and unusual fluid retention, you may be feeling the inflammation of a bladder or kidney infection. A gentle, natural, cleansing course might be just the thing to keep you from getting a full-blown, painful bladder infection.

Kidney function is vital to health. The kidneys are largely responsible for the elimination of waste products from protein breakdown (such as urea and ammonia). If the movement of salts, proteins or other biochemicals goes awry, a whole range of health problems arises, from mild water retention to major kidney failure, and mineral loss. Concentrated protein wastes can cause chronic inflammation of the kidney's filtering tissues (nephritis), and overload the bloodstream with toxins, causing uremia.

But your bladder and kidneys do more than just remove water wastes. They are part of a complex process that maintains body fluid stability. Urinary controls are involved with the brain, hormones, and receptors all over the body. They are smart controls that register what your body needs in the way of fluids. So sometimes they remove very little salt or water, at other times they remove a lot.

A bladder and kidney cleanse is simple, and usually works right away. A three to five day cleanse can often clear out toxic infection quickly.
•Each morning take 2 TBS. cider vinegar or lemon juice in water. Take one each of the following juices each day of the cleanse:

> carrot/beet/cucumber
> unsweetened cranberry
> a mixed vegetable juice
> a green drink such as the one on the next page

•Mid-morning, take a cup of the following green tea herbal cleanser: BANCHA LF., BURDOCK RT., KUKICHA TWIG, GOTU KOLA, FO TI RT., HAWTHORN BRY., ORANGE PEEL CINNAMON BK., ORANGE BLOSSOM OIL. (CD - 6400) *Note:* Continue with a morning green drink or the green tea cleanser for the rest of the month.

•Drink 6 extra glasses of bottled water each day of the cleanse.
•After the three days, add sea foods and sea vegetables, whole grains and vegetable proteins. Eat simply prepared, low salt, low protein, vegetarian foods with 75% in fresh produce. (This type of diet should also be followed for the two weeks after your cleanse for best results.)
•Long term kidney healing foods include garlic and onions, papayas, bananas, watermelon, sprouts, leafy greens and cucumbers. Take some of these frequently during the rest of the month.

Here are some brief pointers to give you the best results for your kidney cleanse:

✓The night before you begin, take a bladder-cleansing herb tea, like the one below: **Uva Ursi Lf., Juniper Bry. & Oil, Corn Silk, Parsley Lf., Dandelion Lf., Plantain Lf., Ginger Rt. & Oil, Cleavers Herb, Marshmallow Rt.** (cd - 5020). This tea may also be used throughout your cleanse. Add $1/4$ teasp. ascorbate C crystals to the tea every time you take it.

✓Avoid dietary irritants on the kidneys, such as coffee, alcohol, and excessive protein.

✓Avoid heavy starches, red and prepared meats, dairy products (except yogurt or kefir), refined, salty, fatty and fast foods for at least a month during healing. They all inhibit kidney filtering.

✓Apply wet, hot compresses on the lower back to speed cleansing; or take alternating hot and cold sitz baths.

✓Take hot saunas to release toxins and excess fluids, and to flush acids out through the skin.

✓Herbal supplements provide excellent support for a kidney cleanse. Take them as liquids, mixed into water or juice, for best results. A superfood green supplement, like the one below is highly recommended:

Rice Protein, Barley Grass & Sprouts, Alfalfa Leaf & Sprouts, Bee Pollen, Acerola Cherry, Oat & Quinoa Sprouts, Apple Pectin, Siberian Ginseng Rt., Sarsaparilla, Spirulina, Chlorella, Dandelion Rt. & Lf., Dulse, Licorice Rt., Gotu Kola Lf. (sa - 8150)

✓Naturopaths emphasize the importance of ample, high-quality water for kidney health. Dehydration is the most common stress on the kidneys. Body purification systems operate efficiently only if the volume of water flowing through them is sufficient to carry away wastes. Drink 6 to 8 glasses of water or other cleansing fluids daily for kidney health.

Note: For kidney stones, see OLIVE OIL FLUSHES under the Liver Cleansing Liquid Diet in this booklet, or. the KIDNEY STONES chapter in HEALTHY HEALING by Linda Rector Page.

See **HEALTHY HEALING** or **COOKING FOR HEALTHY HEALING** by Linda Rector Page for complete bladder and kidney diets and details.

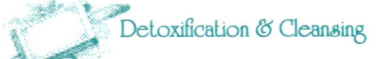

Mucous Congestion Cleanse: *a 3 to 7 day liquid diet.*

A lung and mucous congestion cleanse can help if you have chronic colds, allergies or asthma. We tend to think of body mucous as a bad thing. But the same mucous, that obstructs our breathing during a sinus infection, asthma or a cold, also protects our tissues.

Human beings take about 22,000 breaths a day, and along with the oxygen, we take in dirt, pollen, disease germs, smoke and other pollutants. Mucous gathers up these irritants as they enter the nose and throat, protecting the mucous membranes that line the upper respiratory system. Excess mucous may be a sign that the body is trying to bring itself to health.

The body works together. Extra pressure of disease or heavy elimination on one part of the body puts extra stress on another. Support for the kidneys, for example, takes part of the waste elimination load off the lungs so they can recover faster. Similarly, promoting respiratory health also helps digestive and skin cleansing problems. The lungs, though, are on the front line of toxic intake from viruses, allergies, pollutants, and mucous-forming congestants.

Here are some brief pointers to give you the best results for your excess mucous cleanse:

✓Herbal supplements are a good choice for a mucous congestion cleanse. They act as premier broncho-dilators and anti-spasmodics to open congested airspaces. They can soothe bronchial inflammation and cough. They have the ability to break up mucous. They are expectorants to remove mucus from the lungs and throat.

✓Drink 8 to 10 glasses of healthy liquids daily to thin mucous and aid elimination.

✓Take 10,000mg ascorbate vitamin C crystals with bioflavonoids daily the first three days; just dissolve $1/_4$ teasp. in water or juice throughout the day, until the stool turns soupy, and tissues are flushed. Take 5,000mg daily for the next four days.

✓Take a brisk, daily walk on each day of your cleanse. Breathe deep to help lungs eliminate mucous.

✓Take an enema the first and last day of your fasting diet to thoroughly clean out excess mucous.

✓Apply wet ginger/cayenne compresses to the chest to increase circulation and loosen mucous.

✓Take a hot sauna or a long warm bath with a rubdown, to stimulate circulation.

✓Use organically grown fresh fruits and vegetables for all juices if possible.

A program to overcome any chronic respiratory problem is usually more successful when begun with a short mucous elimination diet. This allows the body to rid itself first of toxins and accumulations that cause congestion before an attempt is made to change eating habits.

The following diet is an effective example of a 3 to 7 day liquid fast for detoxification. Elimination will begin as soon as the first meal is missed.

The night before....

•Have a small fresh salad with plenty of intestinal "sweepers and scourers," such as beets, celery, cabbage, broccoli, parsley, carrots, etc.

•Mash several garlic cloves and a large slice of onion in a bowl. Stir in 3 TBS. of honey. Cover, and let macerate for 24 hours, then remove garlic and onion and take only the honey/syrup infusion - 1 tsp. 3x daily.

The next day....

On rising: take 2 squeezed lemons in water with 1 TB. maple syrup

Breakfast: take a glass of grapefruit, pineapple, or cranberry juice

Mid-morning: have a glass of *fresh* carrot juice with 1 teasp. Bragg's LIQUID AMINOS added; or a congestion clearing tea like the one below. MA HUANG HERB, LICORICE RT., PLEURISY RT., MULLEIN LF., ROSE HIPS, MARSH-MALLOW RT., PEPPERMINT LF. & OIL, FENNEL SD. & OIL, BONESET HERB, GINGER RT. & OIL, CALENDULA FLR., STEVIA HERB. (B - 5930)

Lunch: have a mixed vegetable juice, like V-8, or a bowl of miso soup with sea veggies snipped on top.

Mid-afternoon: have a superfood drink like the one on page 12 of this booklet), or a tea which aids in oxygen uptake like the one below: FENUGREEK SD., HYSSOP, HOREHOUND, GINKGO BILOBA., ROSE HIPS, MA HUANG, MARSHMALLOW RT., BONESET , ANISE SD., PEPPERMINT LF., WILD CHERRY BK., LOBELIA, STEVIA. (B - 6020)

Supper: take a glass of apple juice or papaya/pineapple juice.

Before retiring: take another cup of hot miso broth with 1 teasp. Bragg's LIQUID AMINOS added for relaxation and strength.

To break your fasting cleanse....

Have a small fresh salad on the last night of the cleanse. Eat small, simple meals the next day. Have toasted wheat germ or muesli, or whole grain granola for your first morning of solid food, with a little yogurt, apple, or pineapple juice. Take a fresh salad for lunch with lemon/oil dressing. Have a fresh fruit smoothie during the day. Fix a baked potato and a light soup or salad for dinner. Avoid pasteurized dairy foods, starchy and refined foods that are a breeding ground for congestion.

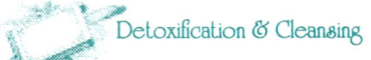

Liver Cleanse: *a 3 day liquid diet.*

Be good to your liver! Your life depends on it. The health and vitality of the entire body depends to a large extent on the health and vitality of the liver. It is the body's most complex organ - a powerful chemical plant that converts everything we eat, breathe and absorb through the skin into life-sustaining substances. The liver is a major blood reservoir, forming and storing red blood cells, and filtering toxins at a rate of a quart of blood per minute. Blood flows directly from the gastrointestinal tract to the liver, so it can neutralize or alter some of the toxic substances before they are distributed to the rest of the body through the blood. Blood also keeps returning to the liver, processing toxins again and again until they are excreted by the bile or kidneys.

A healthy liver can deal with a wide range of toxic chemicals, drugs, solvents, pesticides and food additives. With the acknowledgment that most of us are continually assailed by toxins in our food, water and air, it is generally realized that none of us has a truly healthy liver. The good news is that the liver has amazing rejuvenative powers, and continues to function when as many as 80% of its cells are damaged. Even more remarkable, the liver can regenerate its own damaged tissue.

A liver and organ cleanse can get to the bottom of a lot of health problems. A clean liver is vital for the body to even begin to heal itself. I recommend a short liver cleanse and detoxification twice a year in the spring and fall, using the extra vitamin D from the sun to help. See the liver health pages in **HEALTHY HEALING** by Linda Rector page if your liver is seriously toxic. A complete liver renewal program can take from three to six months.

Do you need a liver cleanse?

Body signals that your liver needs some TLC include unexplained fatigue, weight gain, depression or lethargy, mental confusion, sluggish elimination, food and chemical sensitivities, PMS, jaundiced skin and/or liver spots on the skin, repeated nausea, dizziness and dry mouth.

Here are some brief pointers for the best results in a detox program for liver health:

•Take the strain off your liver by eliminating red meats, refined sugars, preservatives, food dyes and additives. Reducing dietary fat is crucial for liver health and regeneration.

•Eat plenty of vegetables. Have a green, leafy salad every day.

•Drink six to eight glasses of bottled water every day to encourage maximum flushing of liver tissues.

21

•Good liver function depends on the amount and quality of oxygen coming into the lungs. Exercise, air filters, time spent among trees and at the ocean, and early morning sunlight are important.

•Make a point to get adequate rest and sleep during a liver cleanse. The liver does some of its most important work while you sleep!

Here is a liquid 3 day liver cleanse and detoxification diet:

On rising: take 2 TBS. cider vinegar in water with 1 teasp. honey.

Breakfast: take a glass of carrot/beet/cucumber juice, or organic apple juice.

Mid-morning: take a glass of juice with 1 rounded tablespoon of your favorite green superfood mix, or a system-strengthening, nutritionally powerful broth like the one below:

Herbs: ALFALFA LF., BORAGE SD., YELLOW DOCK RT., OATSTRAW, DANDELION LF., BARLEY GRASS, LICORICE RT., WATERCRESS LF., PAU D'ARCO BK., NETTLES HERB, HORSETAIL, RED RASPBERRY, FENNEL SD, PARSLEY RT. & LF., BILBERRY, SIBERIAN GINSENG RT., SCHIZANDRA BRY., ROSEMARY, *Sea Vegetables:* DULSE, WAKAME, KOMBU, SEA PALM. Foods: MISO PWD., SOY PROTEIN, TAMARI PWD., CRANBERRY JUICE PWD., NUTRITIONAL YEAST. (SA - 8230)

Lunch: have a glass of organic apple juice or fresh carrot juice.

Mid-afternoon: have a cup of peppermint tea, pau d'arco tea, or a cleansing combination tea to re-establish an alkaline environment:

DANDELION RT., WATERCRESS LF., YELLOW DOCK RT., HYSSOP HERB, PAU D'ARCO BK., PARSLEY LF., OREGON GRAPE RT., RED SAGE, LICORICE RT., MILK THISTLE SD., HIBISCUS FLR., WHITE SAGE OIL, ANISE OIL. (CD- 5780)

Dinner: have another glass of organic apple juice, or another potassium broth.

Before bed: take another glass of lemon juice or cider vinegar in water. Add 1 teasp. honey or royal jelly.

A helpful supplement program accelerates liver detoxification.

Some supplements may affect the cleansing process, I recommend only using the following until after heavy cleansing is over.

•Ascorbate or Ester C vitamin C crystals with bioflavonoids $1/4$ to $1/2$ teasp. at a time in aloe vera juice.

•One teasp. high quality royal jelly added to any cleansing liquids for increased benefits.

•Fifteen MILK THISTLE SEED EXTRACT (CD- 4560) drops in hot water. Milk Thistle contains some of the most potent liver protecting substances known. The components of this herb stimulate protein synthesis, increasing the production of new liver cells to replace damaged old ones.

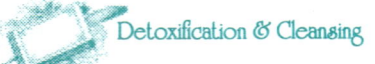

Blood Purifying Cleanse: *a 3 to 7 day diet.*

Your blood is your river of life. The health of your blood is critical. The blood must supply oxygen to the body's sixty trillion cells, transport nutrients, hormones and wastes, warm and cool the body, ward off invading micro-organisms, seal off wounds and much more. It is the chief neutralizing agent for bacteria and toxic wastes. Many diseases are the result of blood toxins. Although not immediately obvious, environmental toxins ingested in sub-lethal amounts can eventually set the environment for disease. Slow viruses that lead to nerve diseases like M.S. can enter the cells and remain dormant for years, mutating and feeding on toxic substances, then reappear in a more dangerous form. While the body has its own self-purifying complex for maintaining healthy blood, the best way to protect yourself from disease is to keep those cleansing systems in good working order.

Here are some of the reasons you might need a blood cleanse:

1) Heavy metal poisoning has become a major health problem of modern society. Numerous studies indicate a strong relationship between heavy metal storage in the body, childhood learning disabilities and criminal behavior. If you served in Vietnam, if your work puts you in contact with petro-chemicals, if you live near a congested highway, or in a crop-dusting fly-way, check yourself for the following symptoms of heavy metal/ chemical toxicity:

- a deep, choking cough
- depression, memory loss and unusual insomnia
- schizophrenic behavior, seizures, periodic black-outs
- sexual dysfunction
- black spots on the gums, bad breath/body odor, unusual, severe reactions to foods and odors
- loss of hand/eye coordination, especially in driving

Include daily in your diet to release heavy metals....

Brown rice, miso soup, a glass of aloe vera juice and a glass of fresh carrot juice. Include artichokes to promote the flow of bile, the major pathway for chemical release from the liver. High sulphur foods like garlic, onions and beans are important. Other foods should be organically grown as much as possible.

Do not go on an all-liquid diet to release heavy metals or chemicals from the body. They enter the bloodstream too fast and heavily for the body to handle, and will poison you even more.

An effective herbal remedy course should include ECHINACEA ROOT extract or PAU D' ARCO/ECHINACEA extract, 3 times daily to cleanse the lymph glands, a superfood green drink such as chlorella or spirulina, or the green drink on page 12. and an herbal compound to help neutralize and release hazardous chemicals that looks like this:

ASCORBATE VIT. C POWDER, BLADDERWRACK, KELP, BUGLEWEED, ASTRAGALUS RT., BARLEY GRASS, PRICKLY ASH, LICORICE RT., PARSLEY RT. (CD - 2450)

A strong, accompanying supplement program should include antioxidants like OPCs from grape seed or pine bark extract, Co-Q$_{10}$, beta-carotene, vitamin C (5 to 10,000mg. daily), and cysteine, a heavy metal chelator.

See HEAVY METAL POISONING, page 387 in Healthy Healing Tenth Edition by Linda Rector Page for more detailed information.

2) Serious immune compromised diseases can benefit from a blood purifying cleanse to boost immune response. There is usually a great deal of blood toxicity, fatigue and lack of nutrient assimilation in serious degenerative conditions like HIV infection, Chronic Fatigue Syndrome, Fibromyalgia, Candidiasis or Lupus. A liquid fast is *not recommended*, since it is often too harsh for an already weakened system. The initial diet should, however, be as pure as possible, in order to be as cleansing as possible - totally vegetarian - free of all meats, dairy foods, fried, preserved and refined foods, and above all, saturated fats. This diet may be followed for 1 to 2 months, or longer if the body is still actively cleansing, or needs further alkalizing. The diet may also be returned to when needed, to purify against relapse or additional symptoms.

Note: A simple blood-color test monitors blood improvement. Make a small, quick, sterilized razor cut on your finger. If the blood is a dark, bluish-purplish color it is not healthy. A bright red color indicates healthy blood.

Here are some brief pointers for the best results in a blood purifying cleanse against immune compromised diseases:
•Produce should be organically grown when possible. Avoid canned, frozen, prepackaged foods, and refined foods with colors, preservatives and flavor enhancers. The investment in a good juicer is well worth it.
•Take a colonic irrigation or enema during your blood cleanse, with 1 tsp. chlorella, spirulina or wheat grass powder dissolved in the water.
•Overheating therapy speeds up metabolism and inhibits replication of invading viruses. See page 178 of Healthy Healing Tenth Edition by Linda Rector Page for details on overheating therapy.

•Take unsweetened mild herb teas and bottled mineral water (6 to 8 glasses) throughout each day, to hydrate, alkalize, and keep the body flushed of toxic wastes. Avoid sodas, artificial drinks, concentrated sugars, and sweeteners. Avoid fried foods of any kind.

•For optimum results, $^1/_2$ teasp. ascorbate vitamin C crystals with bioflavonoids may be added to any blood cleansing drink.

•Sprinkling $^1/_2$ teasp. lactobacillus powder in any juice, or over any cooked food, makes a big difference to your body chemistry change.

•Exercise daily in the morning, if possible. Aerobic oxygen intake alone can be an important nutrient.

Note: See HEALTHY HEALING or COOKING FOR HEALTHY HEALING for complete blood cleansing diets and details.

Vigorous treatment is necessary for immune compromised diseases; supplements are desirable for a blood cleanse against them.

•Anti-oxidants, like germanium 150mg, astragalus extract, vitamin E 1000IU with selenium 200mcg, CoQ_{10} 180mg daily can all strengthen white blood cell and T-cell activity. Quercetin and bromelain help with auto-immune reactions, and offer plant source digestive enzymes.

•Egg yolk lecithin, for active lipids to make cell walls resist attack.

•Acidophilus culture complex with bifidus - refrigerated, highest potency, 3 teasp. daily, with biotin 1000mcg.

•Aloe vera juice concentrate in water daily, to block auto-immune, retro viruses spreading from cell to cell.

•Shark or bovine tracheal cartilage, 740mg, 6 daily.

•ECHINACEA (PD - 4400) OR ECHINACEA/PAU DE ARCO extract (PD- 4570)3x daily, to stimulate production of interferon, interleukin and lymphocytes.

•Carnitine 500mg daily for 3 days. Rest for 7 days, then take 1000mg for 3 days. Rest for 7 days. Take with high Omega-3 fish or flax oils, 3 to 6 daily, and EVENING PRIMROSE OIL 1000mg 3x daily.

A serious blood cleansing program should be accompanied by a serious herbal purifier, especially if you are detoxifying from alcohol or drug overload. The following formula should be taken *without* other supplements for at least 1 month.

RED CLOVER BLSM., LICORICE RT., ASCORBATE VIT. C, BURDOCK RT., PAU D' ARCO BK., SARSAPARILLA RT., KELP, ALFALFA LF., ECHINACEA PURPUREA RT., BUTTERNUT BK., GARLIC, GOLDENSEAL RT., ASTRAGALUS RT., YELLOW DOCK RT., BUCKTHORN BK., PRICKLY ASH BK., PORIA MUSHROOM, AMERICAN PANAX GINSENG RT., DANDELION RT., MILK THISTLE SD. (CD - 2000)

After a serious blood cleanse, an herbal combination to stimulate better circulation, to deter formation and "stickiness" of serum lipids and to maintain arterial blood composition is recommended. The following formula is particularly effective when circulation is sluggish or impeded, and vascular tone is weak. It is rich in absorbable herbal iron. Many people report a tingle in the hands and feet after using this tea as circulation increases to the extremities.

HAWTHORN LF., FLR. & BRY., BILBERRY, KUKICHA TWIG, GINGER RT. & OIL, HEARTSEASE LF., GINKGO BILOBA LF., PAU D' ARCO BK., RED SAGE LF., LICORICE RT., WHITE SAGE & OIL, ASTRAGALUS RT. (CD - 5100)

3) **A program for overcoming addictions and alcohol abuse** reveals far more success when treatment is begun with a blood purifying cleanse. Follow-up studies indicate that as many as 75% of patients are still sober after one year when they first follow a detoxification program. A detox diet is positive support therapy in successful recovery from drug, alcohol, nicotine or concentrated sugar addictions. The overwhelming majority of habitual drug and controlled substance users suffer from malnutrition, metabolic upset and nutritional imbalances. When these conditions are corrected, the need to get high by artificial means is sharply diminished.

Many naturopaths recommend that serious blood cleansing program to overcome addictions be accompanied by a liquid juice diet. Vegetable and fruit juices stimulate rapid, heavy toxin and drug residue elimination, a process that can generate mild symptoms of a "healing crisis." A slight headache, nausea, bad breath, body odor and dark urine occur as the body accelerates release of accumulated toxins. Five to 10,000mg of ascorbate Vitamin C s recommended daily during serious cleansing, to help keep the body alkaline, encourage oxygen uptake, and promote collagen development for new healthy tissue. Vitamin C should be added especially if you are detoxifying from alcohol or drug overload.

The following diet pointers not only helps purify toxic blood, but also help rebuild a depleted system. The diet should be rich in vegetable proteins, high in minerals (especially magnesium for nerve stress), with Omega-3 oils, vitamin B and C source foods, and antioxidants. Regeneration takes time....sometimes up to a year to detoxify and clear drugs from the blood.

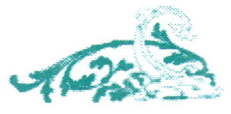

Here are some brief diet pointers for the best results in a detox program to overcome addictions:

•Eat magnesium-rich foods - green leafy and yellow vegetables, citrus fruits, whole grain cereals, fish, and legumes.

•Eat potassium-rich foods - oranges, broccoli, green peppers, seafoods, sea vegetables, bananas, and tomatoes.

•Eat chromium-rich foods, such as brewer's yeast, mushrooms, whole grains, sea foods and peas.

•Eat vegetable protein at every meal. Get some exercise every day.

•Take kudzu caps. Research on kudzu for over-consumption of alcohol shows a reduction in alcohol intake.

•Avoid smoking and secondary smoke. Tobacco increases craving for all drugs.

Herbs provide strengthening support for a blood cleanse to detoxify from alcohol or drugs. Purifying herbs can maintain energy levels and nerve stability during heavy metabolic waste elimination. A good example of a cleansing and purifying herbal tea with this type of activity might look like this:

RED CLOVER , HAWTHORN, HORSETAIL, ECHINACEA PURPUREA LF., MILK THISTLE SD., PAU D' ARCO BK., GOTU KOLA HERB, LEMONGRASS & OIL, BLUE MALVA FLR., YERBA SANTA LF. (CD - 5120)

Herbs can also supply concentrated chlorophyll benefits to normalize body chemistry. The molecular composition of chlorophyll is so close to that of human haemoglobin that a series of green drinks is almost like giving yourself a small, purifying transfusion. An herbal green drink or capsules with normalizing properties looks like this:

RICE PROTEIN, BARLEY GRASS AND SPROUTS, ALFALFA LEAF & SPROUTS, BEE POLLEN, ACEROLA CHERRY, OAT & QUINOA SPROUTS, APPLE PECTIN, SIBERIAN GINSENG, SARSAPARILLA, SPIRULINA, CHLORELLA, DANDELION, DULSE, LICORICE RT., GOTU KOLA. (SA - 8150)

Herbs are a proven choice to help overcome drug-related depression during detoxification. Numerous tests show herbal anti-depressants have few almost no side effects and provide long-lasting relief. I recommend a formula that looks like this to be taken on an as-needed basis:

SCULLCAP LF., ASHWAGANDHA RT. & LF., ST. JOHN'S WORT HERB, VALERIAN RT., ROSEMARY LF., HOPS, CATNIP HERB, WOOD BETONY LF., PEPPERMINT LF., CELERY SD., CINNAMON BK. (CO - 4730)

Note: Add EVENING PRIMROSE OIL or high Omega-3 flax oil when taking this formula to stimulate prostaglandin balance.

27

Herbs can provide needed body energy to get you through addiction craving while you are detoxifying. They offer metabolic and mental energy without overstimulation. The formula below supplies almost immediate energy of this type:

GOTU KOLA HERB, DAMIANA LF., PEPPERMINT LF. & OIL, RED CLOVER BLOSSOM, PRINCE GINSENG RT., KAVA KAVA RT., ARALIA RT., RED RASPBERRY LF., CLOVES FRUIT & OIL. (E - 5570)

Additional supplements to help overcome addictions:

•Take antioxidants like vitamin C crystals, 5 to 10,000mg, in water 3x daily, (or til bowel movement turns soupy) as a detoxifying agent, and vitamin E to strengthen adrenals and restore liver function.

•Take Stress B Complex daily, 150mg for balance.

•Consider a withdrawal support herbal formula that looks like this:

SCULLCAP, SIBERIAN GINSENG RT., VIT. C POWDER, KAVA KAVA RT., VALERIAN RT., ALFALFA, WOOD BETONY, DLPA 35MG, NIACIN 35MG, LICORICE RT., CAPSICUM. (CD - 4330).

Note: Take glutamine 500mg and tyrosine 500mg daily with this formula to help reduce drug cravings.

•Take a full spectrum herbal mineral for system stability. Use every other month to encourage better mineral/nutrient uptake by the body.:

NETTLES, IRISH MOSS, WATERCRESS, ALFALFA, YELLOW DOCK RT., DANDELION RT. & LF., PARSLEY RT. & LF., BARLEY GRASS, KELP, PARSLEY RT. & LF., BORAGE SD., DULSE, L-GLUTAMINE. (SA - 3200)

BODYWORK TECHNIQUES FOR DETOXIFICATION

Detoxification bodywork can accelerate your cleanse. Here are some good choices to work with:

Therapeutic baths: Clinics and spas are famous all over the world for their mineral, seaweed and enzyme baths. The skin is the body's largest organ of ingestion, and can assimilate the valuable nutrients from a therapeutic bath in a pleasant, stress-free way. Bathe at least twice daily during a cleanse to remove toxins coming out through the skin. The procedure for taking an effective healing bath is important. In essence, you are soaking in an herbal tea or mineral fluid, and allowing the skin to take in the healing nutrients instead of the mouth and digestive system.

Here's how: Draw very hot bath water. Put the herbs, seaweeds, or mineral crystals into a large teaball or muslin bath bag. Add mineral salts directly to the water. Steep until water cools and is aromatic. Or, make a strong tea infusion in a large teapot, strain and add to bath water.

•All over dry skin brushing before the bath for 5 minutes with a natural bristle brush will help remove toxins from the skin and open pores for better assimilation of nutrients.

•After the bath, use a mineral salt rub, such as a traditional spa "finishing" technique to make your skin feel healthy for hours:

SUNDRIED SEA SALT, ALOE VERA POWDER, LEMON PEEL GRANULES, ALMOND OIL, LEMON OIL. (BB - 7260)

A hot seaweed bath is a great way to accelerate detoxification.

Seaweed baths are Nature's perfect body/psyche balancer. Remember how good you feel after a walk in the ocean? Seaweeds purify and balance the ocean; they can do the same for your body. Noticeable rejuvenating effects occur when toxins are released from your tissues. A hot seaweed bath is like a wet-steam sauna, only better, because the sea greens normalize body chemistry instead of dehydrating it. The electrolytic magnetic action of the seaweed releases excess body fluids from congested cells, and dissolves fatty wastes through the skin, replacing them with depleted minerals, particularly potassium and iodine. And because iodine boosts thyroid activity, food fuels are used before they can turn into fatty deposits. Vitamin K in seaweeds aids adrenal regulation, meaning that a seaweed bath can help maintain hormone balance for a more youthful body.

Gathering your own seaweed is time-consuming and cumbersome.... even if you live near an ocean.. Crystal Star Herbal Nutrition packages quality dried seaweeds, gathered from the San Juan Islands, in a made-to-order HOT SEAWEED BATH.

KELP, KOMBU, BLADDERWRACK, DULSE, SEA GRASSES. (CD - 7220)

Hot and cold hydrotherapy helps open and stimulate the body's vital healing energies. Alternating hot and cold showers, are effective for getting the body started on a positive track toward healing. Spasmodic pain and cramping, circulation, muscle tone, bowel and bladder problems, system balance, and energy all show improvement with hydrotherapy.

•Begin with a comfortably hot shower for three minutes. Follow with a sudden change to cold water for 2 minutes. Repeat this cycle three times, ending with cold. Follow with a full or partial massage, or a brisk towel rub and mild stretching exercises for best results.

About the Author....

L inda Rector Page has been working in the fields of nutrition and herbal medicine both professionally and as a personal lifestyle choice, since the early seventies. She is a certified Doctor of Naturopathy and Ph.D., with extensive experience in formulating and testing herbal combinations. She received a Doctorate of Naturopathy from the Clayton School of Holistic Healing in 1988, and a Ph.D. in Nutritional Therapy from the American Holistic College of Nutrition in 1989. She is a member of both the American and California Naturopathic Medical Associations.

Linda opened and operated the "Rainbow Kitchen," a natural foods restaurant, then became a working partner in The Country Store Natural Foods store. She has written four successful books and a Library Series of specialty books in the nutritional healing field. Today, she lectures around the country and in the media on a wide range of natural healing topics.

Linda is the founder and formulator of Crystal Star Herbal Nutrition, a manufacturer of over 250 premier herbal compounds. A major, cutting edge influence in the herbal medicine field, Crystal Star Herbal Nutrition products are carried by over twenty-five hundred natural food stores in the U.S. and around the world.

Continuous research in all aspects of the alternative healing world has been the cornerstone of success for her reference work *Healthy Healing* now in its tenth edition. Feedback from all these sources provides up-to-the-minute contact with the needs, desires and results being encountered by people taking more responsibility for their own health. Much of the lifestyle information and empirical observation detailed in her books comes from this direct experience.

Cooking For Healthy Healing, now in its second revised edition, is a companion to Healthy Healing. It draws on both the recipes from the Rainbow Kitchen and the more defined, lifestyle diets that she has developed for healing since then. The book contains thirty-three diet programs, and over 900 healthy recipes.

In *How To be Your Own Herbal Pharmacist*, Linda addresses the rising appeal of herbs and herbal healing in America. This book is designed for those wishing to take more definitive responsibility for their health through individually developed herbal combinations.

Linda's newest work is a party reference book called *Party Lights*, written with restaurateur and chef Doug Vanderberg. *Party Lights*, takes healthy cooking one step further by adding in the fun to a good diet.

Published by Healthy Healing Publications, 1996.

About This Booklet

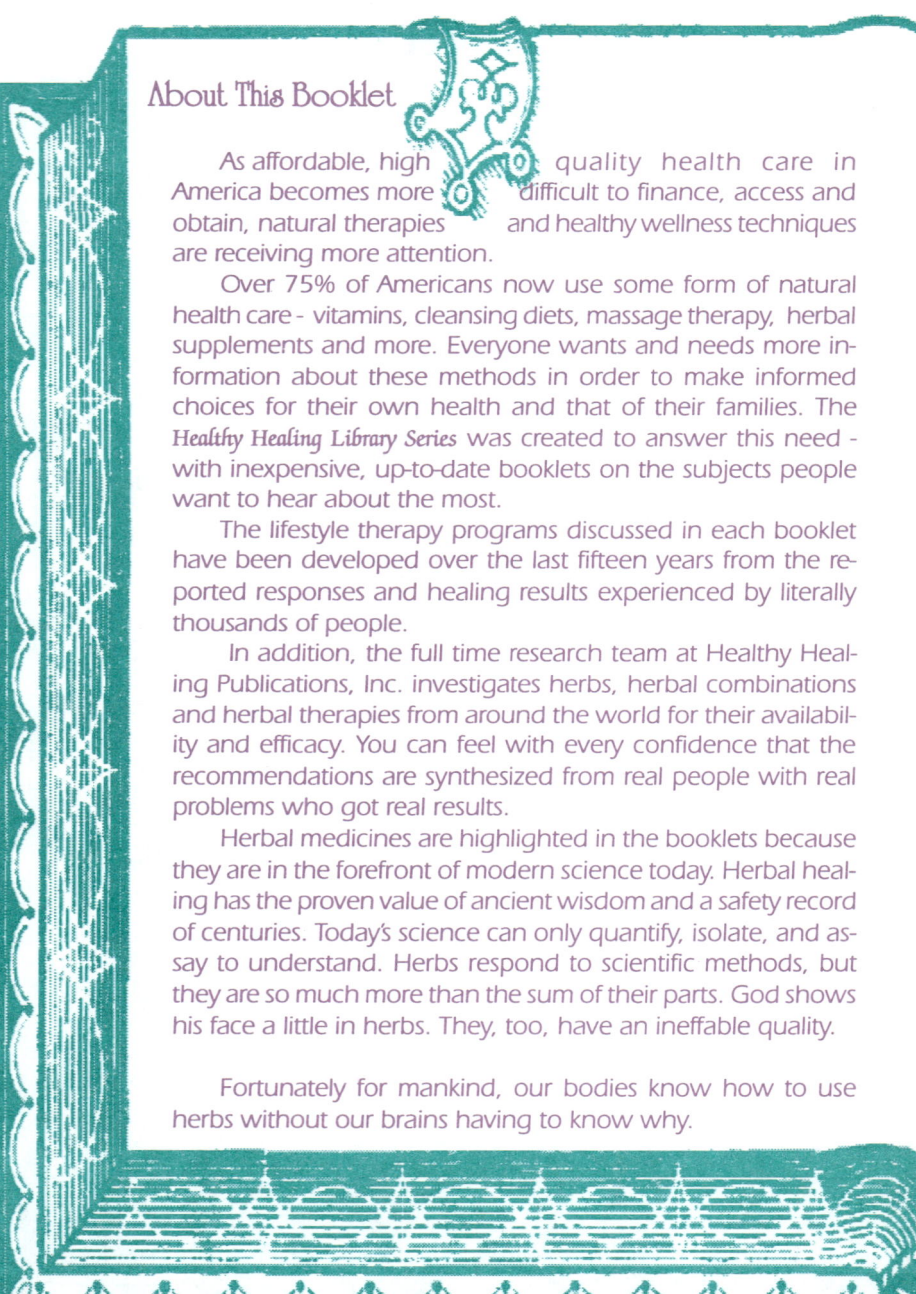

As affordable, high quality health care in America becomes more difficult to finance, access and obtain, natural therapies and healthy wellness techniques are receiving more attention.

Over 75% of Americans now use some form of natural health care - vitamins, cleansing diets, massage therapy, herbal supplements and more. Everyone wants and needs more information about these methods in order to make informed choices for their own health and that of their families. The *Healthy Healing Library Series* was created to answer this need - with inexpensive, up-to-date booklets on the subjects people want to hear about the most.

The lifestyle therapy programs discussed in each booklet have been developed over the last fifteen years from the reported responses and healing results experienced by literally thousands of people.

In addition, the full time research team at Healthy Healing Publications, Inc. investigates herbs, herbal combinations and herbal therapies from around the world for their availability and efficacy. You can feel with every confidence that the recommendations are synthesized from real people with real problems who got real results.

Herbal medicines are highlighted in the booklets because they are in the forefront of modern science today. Herbal healing has the proven value of ancient wisdom and a safety record of centuries. Today's science can only quantify, isolate, and assay to understand. Herbs respond to scientific methods, but they are so much more than the sum of their parts. God shows his face a little in herbs. They, too, have an ineffable quality.

Fortunately for mankind, our bodies know how to use herbs without our brains having to know why.

Bibliography & Other Reading

Rector Page, Linda. *Healthy Healing, Tenth Edition*. 1996

Jensen, Bernard, D.C., Nutritionist. *Tissue Cleansing Through Bowel Management*. 1981

Cassata, Carla. "How To Balance Body Chemistry." *Let's Live*. March 1995

Hobbs, Christopher. "Herbs For Health - Losing Addictions Naturally." *Let's Live*. April 1993

Benninger, Jon. "Detox." *The Energy Times*. July 1994

Thomson, Bill. "Rejuvenate Yourself in Three Weeks." *Natural Health*. January 1993

Langer, Stephen, M.D. "Keeping Environmental Toxins At Bay," *Better Nutrition For Today's Living*. July 1993

Hobbs, Christopher. "Tonics, Bitters, Digestion, and Elimination." *Let's Live*. August 1990

Goldberg, Burton. "Detoxification Therapy." *Alternative Medicine - The Definitive Guide*. 1993

Larson, Joan Mathews, Ph.D. *Seven Weeks To Sobriety*. 1992

Schechter, Steven R., N.D. *Fighting Radiation & Chemical Pollutants With Foods, Herbs & Vitamins* - Documented Natural Remedies That Boost Your Immunity & Detoxify.

Booklets
in the
Library Series

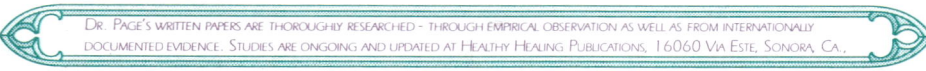

DR. PAGE'S WRITTEN PAPERS ARE THOROUGHLY RESEARCHED - THROUGH EMPIRICAL OBSERVATION AS WELL AS FROM INTERNATIONALLY DOCUMENTED EVIDENCE. STUDIES ARE ONGOING AND UPDATED AT HEALTHY HEALING PUBLICATIONS, 16060 VIA ESTE, SONORA, CA.,